Yogi cats

Paige Hodges

PASSION
FRUIT
PRESS

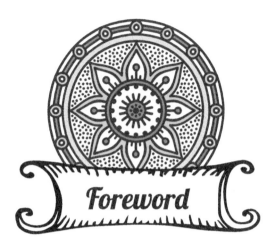

Foreword

By Paige Hodges

As a young adult living in New York City, a mouse sighting in my small studio apartment left me a bit unsettled. "Get a cat," a friend said, "and you'll never have to worry about mice again." So I did and thus my love affair with the feline species began! A few years later, my three cats and I moved to Los Angeles, CA. Shortly after my arrival, my friend, Judith, took me to a yoga class for my birthday and I was immediately hooked! Thus my love affair with yoga began!

Yoga and cats are a huge part of my life. I have been practicing yoga for well over 20 years and credit my practice with giving me balance in all areas of my life. I have had the honor to study with some of the world's best Iyengar yoga teachers and to serve on the Board of the Iyengar Yoga Association of Los Angeles. No matter one's age or physical condition, I believe that yoga has something to offer us all.

Wanting to merge my love of yoga and cats, I founded Feline Yogi, a company that makes yoga mats just for kitties. In addition to my "catepreneur" endeavors, I have worked and volunteered for several local Los Angeles-based cat welfare organizations and I'm a strong advocate of spay/neuter and Trap Neuter Return Programs (TNR) for cats. I am passionate about ending the cat overpopulation problem so that no cats are ever killed due to lack of homes or space in shelters.

Yoga and cats complement each other purr-fectly! Yoga practice gives us strength, stamina, balance, and flexibility. Cats are soothing to our spirit and their energy makes us feel at ease. A cat's presence commands attention and you automatically gravitate towards wanting to spend time with them. Cats have a great deal to teach us about yoga and having a cat in your life is like having your own personal guru. A guru you have to feed and whose litter box needs scooping, but nevertheless, a world class guru!

Felines are the original yoga practitioners. Their limber bodies and generally relaxed, natural dispositions enable them to fall into a deep meditative state—the goal of yoga asana practice. Cats have perfected Shavasana (resting pose) and practice it numerous times throughout the day. Cats are accepting of their bodies and understand that we all come in different shapes and sizes and we are all gorgeous. They know that it would be boring if we all had the same body type or fur pattern.

I am grateful for yoga and for the cats I have known who have taught me so much, especially how to live in the present. Felines know the present is the greatest gift of all and they teach us to indulge in it because the present is all we ever really have.

Meow and Namaste!

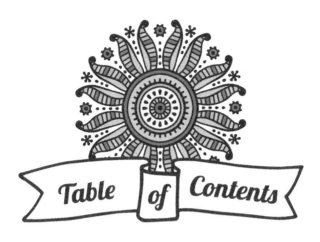

Table of Contents

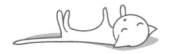

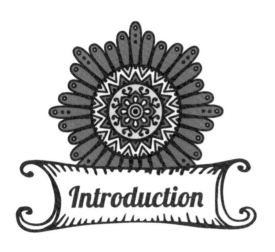

Introduction

From their feline grace and agility to their relaxed nature, cats should be every yogi's influence as they pray om with each yoga position. Whether you are a novice in the art of yoga or a veteran yogi, no doubt you can appreciate the serene nature of spiritual reflection next to your adorable kitty cat. There are times to laze around like a cat in the sun and there are times to be as playful as a kitten in a basket of yarn, so whatever inspiration you're looking for to compliment your yogi wishes, look no further than your kitty companion.

If you love yoga and cats, then you're about to live in purrfect harmony.

Breath

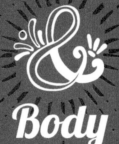

Body

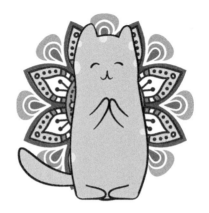

Lotus Pose

Sit down on the ground and calmly cross your legs. Put your right foot on your left thigh as close to your groin as you can. Put your left foot on your right thigh, but be careful not to lose your balance. Lay your hands freely over your knees. If you want more stability, you may push your palms against the floor to keep you centered. Take even breaths and hold.

"We are aware of yoga only as a technique to gain physical strength, flexibility, or increased health. And indeed these are potent side effects of the practice. But that is what they are: side effects. To focus on these largely insignificant manifestations is to miss the point entirely."

John McAfee

Your body is a temple and inside holds your spirit. Practicing yoga is the gateway to healing your body. Just as how cats do a routine cleansing of their bodies, yoga is the routine cleansing of your mind, to purge out toxins and take in positivity. You will open your heart to a spiritual awakening with daily practice, and you will learn the beauty of patience and contemplation.

"When the breath wanders, the mind also is unsteady. But when the breath is calmed, the mind too will be still, and the yogi achieves long life. Therefore, one should learn to control the breath."

Hatha Yoga Pradipika

Taking deep, calm breaths will steady your heart. Outside elements may cause you to get anxious, stressed, and angry, but when you take a moment to release that negativity through even breaths, you will never find yourself gasping for air. Calm your breathing with your feline companion, taking slow, deep breaths with every purr.

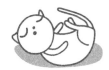

"When you inhale, you are taking the strength from God. When you exhale, it represents the service you are giving to the world."

B.K.S. Iyengar

Every breath you take gives you life and every breath you give feeds life. Find solace in the fact that your existence serves a purpose in the cycle of life and relish in the spiritual connection between you, God, and nature. If you weren't here, then who would snuggle with your kitten every night?

"Yoga practice can make us more and more sensitive to subtler and subtler sensations in the body. Paying attention to and staying with finer and finer sensations within the body is one of the surest ways to steady the wandering mind."

Ravi Ravindra

As the muscles in your body get stronger, so do the muscles in your brain. Just as your tendons tighten to gain maximum strength, your concentration sharpens, like a cat ready to pounce. Focusing on the minute details of your body can translate into focusing on the details of your life. Learn which areas need work to grow, which areas need rest to build, and which areas are ready for challenges.

"The autonomic nervous system is divided into the sympathetic system, which is often identified with the fight-or-flight response, and the parasympathetic, which is identified with what's been called the relaxation response. When you do yoga—the deep breathing, the stretching, the movements that release muscle tension, the relaxed focus on being present in your body—you initiate a process that turns the fight-or-flight system off and the relaxation response on. That has a dramatic effect on the body. The heartbeat slows, respiration decreases, blood pressure decreases. The body seizes this chance to turn on the healing mechanisms."

Richard Faulds

When you take on the challenge of healing your body with yoga, you begin the process of conditioning your body to release the tensions of the world and relax. The hardships and aches in your back, the constriction of your chest, the soreness of your untrained limbs—these will all disappear as you heal yourself from the pains of life. It is good to relax. A cat stays limber from healthy resting.

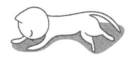

"As I explore the wilderness of my own body, I see that I am made of blood and bones, sunlight and water, pesticide residues and redwood humus, the fears and dreams of generations of ancestors, particles of exploded stars."

Anne Cushman

Discover the miracle that is your existence. You are a collection of generational history, natural beauty, and creative genius, and you should take joy in your being! Meditate on your dreams and conquer your fears. As you discover yourself, gaze at your spirit and awe in admiration of where you come from. You are purrfection!

"Your hand opens and closes and opens and closes. If it were always a fist or always stretched open, you would be paralyzed. Your deepest presence is in every small contracting and expanding, the two as beautifully balanced and coordinated as bird wings."

Rumi

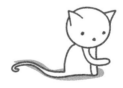

You can read someone's life story in the palm of their hands. The movements of our hands express our state in life, opening and closing opportunities and obstacles as we age. Accept the shifts in life for the lessons they teach with feline agility and grace, or you will be paralyzed by anger and discontent. Hold your hand to your heart and keep yourself balanced.

"Fear less, hope more; eat less, chew more; whine less, breathe more; talk less, say more; hate less, love more; and all good things are yours."

Swedish Proverb

Live life to the fullest. Ridding yourself of unnecessary fears and hatred will cleanse your soul, taking the time to enjoy the food you eat and the conversation you have with loved ones will build memories to cherish. Learning to love the world and let negativity fall off you will bring you happiness. Unlike cats, you do not have nine lives, so make the best of the one you have!

"To keep the body in good health is a duty, otherwise we shall not be able to keep our mind strong and clear."

Buddha

If being healthy was as natural as breathing, then no one would suffer from illness. Keeping good health is a matter of tending to one's own garden, in that the duty of having a disciplined routine will let your body grow ripe with age. Daily caretaking will keep your mind from becoming lazy and uninspired.

"You pray for good health and a body that will be strong in old age. Good—but your rich foods block the gods' answer and tie Jupiter's hands."

Persius

In order to maintain good health, you must do more than pray and wish upon a star. You will need to instill the proper discipline to take care of your body. Be as meticulous as a cat that cleans itself after each foreign contact. Every journey needs nourishment, and as yoga ties you closer to your soul, your diet should tie you closer to a well-nourished body. Be aware of what you take inside.

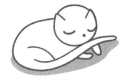

Maintaining your health means fighting constant temptations. Whether you have a sweet tooth or are a victim to junk food, you must face your vices and discipline your desires. It will be hard in the beginning, but eliminating toxins from your body will give you more energy and life. It's okay to treat yourself, but don't lend yourself to becoming a fat cat.

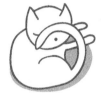

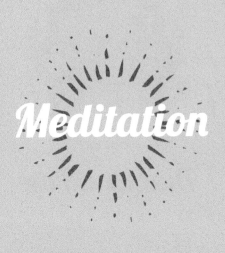

Meditation

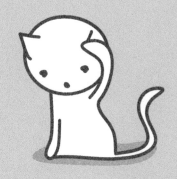

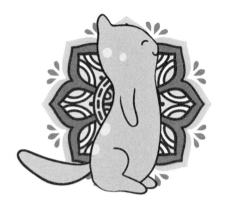

Diamond Pose

Sit on your heels with your back straight. Keep your chin leveled and look forward. Rest your hands on your thighs and take even breaths. Hold this position as you meditate.

"Yoga is the practice of quieting the mind."

Patanjali

As the anxieties and stress of the day begin to overwhelm you, let yoga be the method to quiet them down and give you time to reflect and then focus on the future. Meditation can clear the way for answers and reveal that taking time to relax means solutions are available. When the mind gets too loud, let yoga purr it back to peace.

"The aim of yoga is to eliminate the control that material nature exerts over the human spirit, to rediscover through introspective practice what the poet T.S. Eliot called 'the still point of the turning world.'"

Barbara Stoler Miller

You cannot control outside forces, but you can control yourself. Understanding your spirit as a solid foundation that you can form and mature, you can brace yourself against the overwhelming material temptations and stresses life sends your way. You will have to fight battles, but you do not have to surrender yourself to them. Yoga will give you your own set of claws.

"In this fast-paced, constantly moving world, practicing yoga allows me time to stop and just be aware of where I am and how I feel. It is a time to be one with my body, and let go of all the distractions and worries of the outside world. Holding an asana like Warrior One, with my legs stretched in a lunge and my arms reaching up, I feel grounded and free at the same time. I can sense my body acting as a conduit between the earth and the sky, and feel my breath flowing with this sacred energy."

Jonathan Urla

Take the time to meditate in your own presence and appreciate the energy that flows through when you connect with the world. You are the spiritual connection between earth and the skies, and your body is a channel of positive and negative energy. Let the good in the world flow through you and the ill flow out.

"Yoga takes us to the present moment, the only place where life exists."

Ellen Brenneman

When you practice yoga, forget about the past. There is nothing you can do to reverse any events or change the results. Live in the moment like a kitten ready to pounce on a better future and leave regret behind. Sometimes, changing your position to get a different point of view is the key to finding a solution.

"We all wish for world peace, but world peace will never be achieved unless we first establish peace within our own minds."

Geshe Kelsang Gyatso

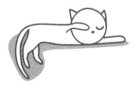

To achieve internal peace, you must have a basis to ground yourself on, principles that will guide you through conflict, forgiveness of your own flaws in order to forgive others, and love for yourself and your dreams so that you will not mock others. Knowing who you are will prevent you from engaging in petty cat fights.

"The affairs of the world will go on forever. Do not delay the practice of meditation."

Milarepa

There will be infinite excuses to prevent yourself from getting into a routine schedule, but if you allow outside forces to mark you a slave to their will instead of yours, then you will never find peace under your terms. You must make time for meditation. If you can make time to laze around with your kitty all day, then imagine how good the snuggles will feel after a good workout

"All of humanity's problems stem from man's inability to sit quietly in a room alone."

Blaise Pascal

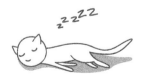

The difficult nature of meditation lies in the act of letting go. With stress about work, relationships, money, and other life challenges, sitting down and meditating might seem like a counterproductive activity in a world of overwhelming priorities. Meditation is about reflection and relief. Like a lion observing its prey, it is the zone in which you attack issues, a successful hunt to feed on good energy.

"Do you have the patience to wait till your mud settles and the water is clear? Can you remain unmoving till the right action arises by itself?"

Tao Te Ching

A disciplined practice you should master as you meditate is the art of patience. Impatience can lead to haste, to reckless actions, to overeager conclusions. Learn to evaluate the situation around you and to take a deep breath before making your next move. The lion cub will strike recklessly and get caught in a trap, but the lioness will wait and kill the zebra when it's time.

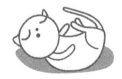

"The witnessing soul is like the sky. The birds fly in the sky, but they don't leave any footprints. That's what Buddha says, that the man who is awakened lives in such a way that he leaves no footprints... He never looks ahead, he never looks back, he lives in the moment."

Osho

People feel the need to find a purpose or leave a legacy that will be remembered for centuries in order to feel important, and they feel worthless when they've produced neither. You were blessed to enjoy this world, to appreciate the beauties it holds, including yourself. Sometimes all that matters is that you soar through this world, giving life and love to those around you.

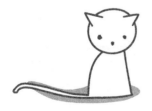

Demons
Inside

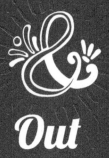

Out

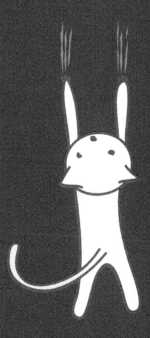

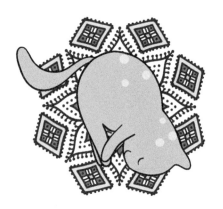

Ragdoll Pose

Take a relaxed stance, exhale and hinge at your hips. As your upper torso relaxes itself into a standing forward bend, allow your knees to bend slightly and your hands to hang loosely, like a rag doll. Let your head hang heavy with your arms to relieve all tensions. Hold here and let your problems wash off of you. Shake your head and arms as if they're particularly large problems.

"The yoga mat is a good place to turn when talk therapy and antidepressants aren't enough."

Amy Weintraub

Yoga is not the cure for everything, but it can be the vitamin or supplement your mind and soul needs. If therapy and medication cannot contain your demons, sometimes it takes a little bit of strength to face them in a mental battle. Yoga can train you to stand against your demons when everything else begins to fade. It can be the extra healing potion in your fight.

"For those wounded by civilization, yoga is the most healing salve."

Terri Guillemets

There is serenity in solitude when you need to restore your spirit with the world. People can be cruel and life can be hard, but instead of letting yourself get consumed by sorrow or anger, channel your negative energy into something productive. While crying with your cat might be one option, let yoga be the sponge to cleanse your wounds so that you can face the world again tomorrow.

"You cannot always control what goes on outside. But you can always control what goes on inside."

Wayne Dyer

Obstacles and hardships will always come; try as you might, there are some things you cannot prevent. Practicing yoga will help you find your center to keep you balanced when the world seems to be in chaos. Stretch your paws up to the skies for answers or keep your feet firmly planted on the ground to keep you level-headed, but always remember you are in control of your mind and body, and thus your place.

"Yoga is about clearing away whatever is in us that prevents our living in the most full and whole way. With yoga, we become aware of how and where we are restricted—in body, mind, and heart—and how gradually to open and release these blockages. As these blockages are cleared, our energy is freed. We start to feel more harmonious, more at one with ourselves. Our lives begin to flow—or we begin to flow more in our lives."

Cybele Tomlinson

When you perform yoga, you must break down your mental barriers. Scratch unneeded worries and restrictions out of your mind, so that you can make choices freely in your pursuit of happiness. It will not be immediate, but as your muscles grow over time, so will your spirit. Knead your anxieties so you can relax, the way a cat kneads a surface before it rests.

"Yoga is really trying to liberate us from shame about our bodies. To love your body is a very important thing—I think the health of your mind depends on your being able to love your body."

Rodney Yee

Strength comes in many forms. The strength of a cat lies in its agility. Yoga allows you to tend to your muscles' growth and the maturation of your spirit, so that you can embrace your own temple in its beauty. You will find grace, balance, and strength in yourself, both physically and mentally, and no longer will you be ashamed to see your own reflection.

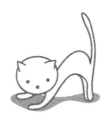

"Warrior pose battles inner weakness and wins focus. You see that there is no war within you. You're on your own side, and you are your own strength."

Terri Guillemets

As you stretch your arms out and feel your muscles begin to quake, focus on the direction your dominant hand points: forward. Notice your body positioned to be on your side, ready for battle, and your legs anchored to give you strength. This is how you approach your dilemmas. You are strong and willing. Let your body be your armor and your mind be your weapon.

"Learning to let go should be learned before learning to get. Life should be touched, not strangled. You've got to relax, let it happen at times, and at others move forward with it."

Ray Bradbury

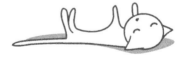

Throughout life, you will learn that nothing is permanent. Moments are as fleeting as a breeze across the grass, present but gone within an instant, but still you enjoy the cool kisses across your cheeks. Learn to let go, to enjoy pleasant times as they come and to remember that hardships are temporary. Value the present and move with it towards a happy future, but do not trick yourself into hanging onto the past.

"All unimportant matters drop off you in ragdoll pose. Very few things are genuinely important. The Truth sways before you."

Terri Guillemets

As you drape your body down to the floor and feel the blood rush through you, let your stress wash off your back. Petty arguments, mild annoyances, tiny grudges—let all of these insignificant poisons fall from your shoulders so that you can breathe deeply without the weight. You do not need them. Instead, say hello to your feline friend reaching up to you, wondering what you're doing.

"If while on your way you meet no one your equal or better, steadily continue on your way alone. There is no fellowship with fools."

Dhammapada

Cats are nice, but catty people aren't. Rid yourself of anyone who only brings negativity your way. This does not mean you should abandon friends who have fallen into despair, but keep wary of people who only wish to drag you into misery with them. Do not disrupt your spiritual journey with an off-course detour to a dead end.

"You only lose what you cling to."

Buddha

Do not let yourself get caught up in worldly possessions. With each meditation you practice, keep all your valuables alive in your concentration: family, friends, and pets. Real bonds that you have with loved ones or your kitties cannot be broken. This union of mind, body, and spirit will keep you together always.

"When you catch yourself slipping into a pool of negativity, notice how it derives from nothing other than resistance to the current situation."

Donna Quesada

Yoga forces you to acknowledge the present situation around you and encourages you to face it, position yourself for it, and embrace it. Whenever you notice yourself beginning a downward spiral, return to yoga as a means to keep you grounded. Like a nimble cat, let yoga twist you around to land on your feet instead of falling into agony.

"Yoga does not remove us from the reality or responsibilities of everyday life, but rather places our feet firmly and resolutely in the practical ground of experience. We don't transcend our lives; we return to the life we left behind in the hopes of something better."

Donna Farhi

Yoga is not an escape from your troubles, but a moment to step back from them and observe where the corrections need to be made. Let meditation be a time of calm, problem-solving and release of anxieties that only inhibit you from taking action. Let the graceful feline motions of your body be expressed in the way you move through life. Take pause and then stretch forward.

"You must purge yourself before finding faults in others. When you see a mistake in somebody else, try to find if you are making the same mistake. This is the way to take [judgment] and to turn it into improvement. Do not look at others' bodies with envy or with superiority. All people are born with different constitutions. Never compare with others. Each one's capacities are a function of his or her internal strength. Know your capacities and continually improve upon them."

B.K.S. Iyengar

More often than not, faults you find in others are also faults you find in yourself. If someone's personality rubs you the wrong way, perhaps they are a slight reflection of your imperfections. If someone's appearance strikes envy or arrogance within you, ask yourself if they are based off insecurities you have of your own body. Rid yourself of any catty thoughts and find the real issue at hand.

"Through practice, I've come to see that the deepest source of my misery is not wanting things to be the way they are. Not wanting myself to be the way I am. Not wanting the world to be the way it is. Not wanting others to be the way they are. Whenever I'm suffering, I find this war with reality to be at the heart of the problem."

Stephen Cope

When you find yourself at odds with your own reality, you must ask yourself why you dislike what you are facing. Instead of pining over what isn't, take solace in what is. Perfection is subjective, an imaginary ideal. What do you find beautiful in others? When you look at your cat, for instance, do you love it for its standard features or the quirks it has? Calm your self-hatred and look inside again. See your beauty.

"Worries are pointless. If there's a solution, there's no need to worry. If no solution exists, there's no point to worry."

Matthieu Ricard

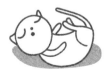

With daily practice, yoga will teach you that worries are worthless. Face your dilemmas with the determination of a cat on the hunt. Focus less on whether you can solve a problem and more on how should you solve a problem. You will live up to the challenge when needed, but in order to do so, you must learn the steps to get there. Have more faith in yourself. If there are solutions, act on them. If there aren't, let go and move on.

"The best fighter is never angry."

Lao Tzu

Anger pollutes your train of thought and blinds you from rational solutions. Never fight when you are consumed by your emotions. Even loved ones will get scratched if the cat is angry. Take a deep breath. Meditate on the problem at hand. Void your body of tension and resentment and stand proud when you are ready. Approach an issue with a level-head and an open mind so that peace can be made.

"Yoga asks you to make peace with the deepest, most terrifying parts of yourself and then make that same peace with the external world."

Kino MacGregor

If you feel uncomfortable sitting quietly with your thoughts, then you are beginning the healing process. You will face your deepest insecurities as you go on this spiritual journey, but as you continue to practice yoga, you will not feel abandoned in your darkness. Instead, the training provided to you by yoga will show a light within your mind to use as a beacon of hope in your spirit.

"The real Meaning of Yoga is a deliverance from contact with pain and sorrow."

Bhagavad Gita

Some people pick up yoga to get into better shape, but most people stay because their mind and spirit have taken on better outlooks. Yoga is the cleansing and routine discipline of keeping the mind from absorbing the negativity in the world. It trains the spirit to wash out demons every day. It teaches the soul to forgive the evil in the world so that it can take in the good.

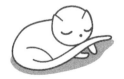

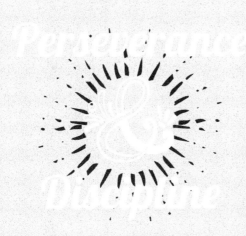

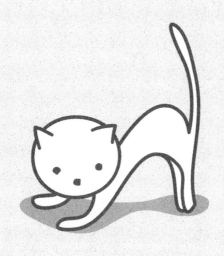

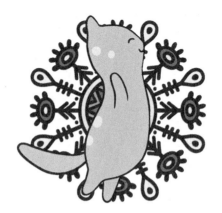

Chair Pose

Stand up straight with your feet apart at shoulder-width. Stretch your arms forward and upon exhale, squat down as low as you can without lifting your heels off the mat. Keep your back straight, as if you were sitting in a chair. You can bend your torso forward to keep you steady. Hold this position. You may keep your arms forward or stretch them up to the sky.

"Our bodies are our gardens—our wills are our gardeners."

William Shakespeare

Your body can possess a strength to challenge the gods, but in order to reach that level, you must tend to your muscles each day with care and observation. Just as how a gardener has different tasks each day for each plant, so should you regard each day for each muscle. Take a lesson from the meticulousness of your cat's daily body maintenance. Respect your body.

"Submit to a daily practice. Your loyalty to that is a ring at the door. Keep knocking, and eventually the joy inside will look out to see who is there."

Rumi

Incorporating yoga into your routine will be an overwhelming struggle at first. You will want to give up or find excuses to push it off, but you must be strict with yourself and find time for a moment of stillness to enter your day. Just as how you find time to take care of your cat's well-being, take time to take care of yours. This dedication will restore peace in your life. When you make your mental stability important, the rest of your day will shape around it.

"Anyone who practices can obtain success in yoga, but not one who is lazy. Constant practice alone is the secret of success."

Svatmarama

If you want to improve yourself, then solely you can provide it. You can't become strong through someone else and you can't find true happiness taking action for others' approval. Yoga is an intimate process, an exercise for the mind, body, and soul. Take yourself seriously and be disciplined.

"You don't have to be flexible to do yoga, you just have to be willing to shake the dust off and see what happens."

David Good

Yoga is a challenging exercise, but it is also an individual challenge worthy of taking on. Whether your flexibility reaches cat-burglar status makes no difference. Going at your own pace is the key to understanding your own challenges. Do not worry about others' levels or battles, and focus on yourself. Your progress is your prize.

"Yoga is like an ocean of wisdom, but we have to go inside to see the beauty of it. An ounce of practice is worth more than tons of theory."

Sharath Rangaswamy

You can only become better once you take action, and you can only stay better if you continue to move. A lion doesn't give up a hunt after missing the first zebra. Even if you can't finish a routine in the beginning or if an injury restrains you from meeting the potential you used to have, by persisting to try and fail, you will get your body to evolve. Practice.

"Stop wondering or regretting, and practice. Yoga teaches us to cure what need not be endured and endure what cannot be cured."

B.K.S. Iyengar

Pain is both a mental and physical factor that you cannot escape from in life, but by incorporating yoga into your routine, you can overcome these battles. Whether you use yoga to soothe your backaches and joint arthritis or as a form of mental rejuvenation in the morning to wash away stress, yoga may be the therapeutic answer to your life.

"Mountain pose is an affirmation. You can conquer anything with your natural boldness and resolute strength. Only you can reach the peak of your success."

Terri Guillemets

In mountain pose, you can stand proudly with your chest out to the world, affirming your existence in the universe. You are important. You are a force to be reckoned with. You are the representation of your own dreams and you are here to achieve them.

"Chair pose is a defiance of spirit, showing how high you can reach even when you're forced down."

Terri Guillemets

Forces in life will attempt to sit you down and keep you subservient, but you're not a dog! You are an independent person with feline grace who must learn to stretch beyond your limits. The first day you perform chair pose, your thighs quake and your weight feels too heavy to bear without tangible support, but with strength training, you will find that the only support you need to achieve anything comes from you and you alone.

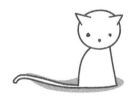

"Usually there's about a three-month love affair with yoga. 'I feel so good.' After about two months of practice, people think they are practically enlightened. Then usually around the third month, something happens and the yoga actually starts to work. And the first thing the ego structure does is to look for an escape route. People start heading for the door just at the moment when they should stay."

Richard Freeman

Everyone reaches a plateau, which can fool you into thinking you have conquered all challenges when you have only conquered the first. Yoga evolves just as you do. Do not shy away from meeting new difficulties to overcome. Approach new challenges the way a cat looks for new heights to leap towards. There are always new platforms to conquer.

"In truth, it matters less what we do in practice than how we do it and why we do it. The same posture, the same sequence, the same meditation with a different intention takes on an entirely new meaning and will have entirely different outcomes."

Donna Farhi

A professional is someone who perfected a task after a million performances of it. Too often people rush to become great at something without putting in the effort to train or noticing their progress along the way. Not every cat landed on its feet the first time it fell. It takes a thousand steps to climb a mountain, so do not look at an exercise as a stifling chore, but as the pathway to perfection.

"Even if things don't unfold the way you expected, don't be disheartened or give up. One who continues to advance will win in the end."

Daisaku Ikeda

Yoga is a test of the spirit. Certain positions will bring you to your knees and others will be moments of relief, but priding yourself in finishing each exercise each day will make it all the worthwhile. With every mountain you climb, the view only gets better. Whether you're straining in Chair Pose or relaxing in Cat Pose, do not give up. Let your inner cat add more moves to its nimbleness.

"Do not ask for less responsibility to be free and relaxed—ask for more strength!"

Shengyan

52

In the beginning, the regimen to abide to will be grueling and you will want to give up halfway, but don't! Cutting yourself short of your duties will not allow you to improve and grow stronger. Do not let yourself become a lazy cat that sleeps all day. What took you an hour to do the first day will take you a minute a few months later. Practice and improve. Let yourself get stronger!

"We are not going in circles, we are going upwards. The path is a spiral; we have already climbed many steps."

Hermann Hesse

What is the point of all your effort if you do the same routine every day? What progress is there to show? Remember that improvement is gradual. Unlike your cat friend, you don't leap to the top, you climb it. Notice the seconds or minutes you shave off your performance. Notice your heart rate grow calmer and your muscles leaner. Small progressions build up to a bigger result.

"One becomes firmly established in practice only after attending to it for a long time, without interruption and with an attitude of devotion."

Yoga Sutra

Some people practice yoga for a month and consider themselves experts, but do not let a sense of arrogance overcome you. It takes years to master the art of yoga, as it ties in with understanding yourself. There are always new lessons and challenges to face. Do not be fooled by playful kittens who just learned how to pounce; it takes time for a cat to learn how to move with grace. Yoga is a lifelong devotion. Do not regard it as a fad.

"Yoga is a light, which once lit, will never dim. The better your practice, the brighter the flame."

B.K.S. Iyengar

No one regrets picking up yoga, but people do regret quitting it. Each session will make your body as flexible as an alley cat, your muscles as strong as a tiger, and your mind as calm as sleeping kitten, but it is imperative that you stick it out. With each day that you fine-tune your body, you will see yourself glow, whether from your healthy skin or your healthy spirit.

Working yoga into your daily routine might seem impossible, especially when life asks many responsibilities of you, but even practicing yoga in the morning for fifteen minutes gives you the perspective of time standing still for you to breathe. Focus on what you need to do, like taking your cat to the vet, but also take a moment to gaze at your life from a distance to feel the quiet peace flow through you.

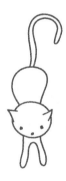

Self-Discovery

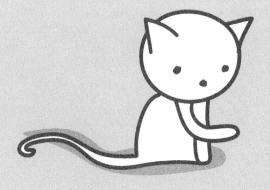

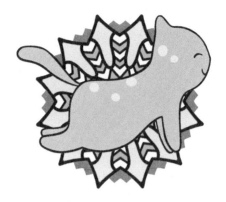

Upward-Facing Dog

Begin by taking the plank pose. Lower your pelvis and thighs close to the ground, keeping your arms straight and your upper body up. Arch your back as you look up to keep your arms and legs try. Aside from your hands and feet, try not to touch the ground with your knees. Hold and breathe deeply.

"Courage is often associated with aggression, but instead should be seen as a willingness to act from the heart."

Donna Quesada

Having courage means to stay true to your principles, to protect those that you care about, to face obstacles for the sake of a better outcome. It does not mean you fight only for domination or with intimidation, like an alpha lion. You fight because you have love to protect and nurture, like a mother lion for her cubs. Fight against the immediate challenges of yoga for your own well-being. Nurture yourself. Love and protect you.

"Every time you are tempted to react in the same old way, ask if you want to be a prisoner of the past, or a pioneer of the future."

Deepak Chopra

Old habits are hard to kill, but the beginning of change is the acceptance that you need to do so. If you are a victim of a poor diet or laziness like a fat cat with cheesy tuna, then ask yourself if you are willing to hate yourself for your choices later or muster up the discipline now and regret nothing. Be your own motivation.

"Don't move the way fear makes you move. Move the way love makes you move. Move the way joy makes you move."

Osho

The journey of your self-discovery should be fueled by the wonderful things you learn about yourself, not focused on insecurities you may have. People preach "embracing imperfection," but you are not imperfect. You were born with lessons to learn, goals to reach, habits to keep. Move in the comfort of your own skin and your being. You are a product of divinity and you have a story of your own!

"Change is not something that we should fear. Rather, it is something that we should welcome. For without change, nothing in this world would ever grow or blossom, and no one in this world would ever move forward to become the person they're meant to be."

B.K.S. Iyengar

It can be scary to start new chapters in your life, especially when you don't have any experience or certainty as to whether you will succeed, but life is a continuous lesson and you should always regard mistakes and failures as part of the learning process. Change can transform you for the greater and your determination will always mold it in your favor. Don't be a scared kitten! Be brave and pounce!

"These days, my practice is teaching me to embrace imperfection: to have compassion for all the ways things haven't turned out as I planned, in my body and in my life— for the ways things keep falling apart, and failing, and breaking down. It's less about fixing things, and more about learning to be present for exactly what is."

Anne Cushman

The world is chaotic and there is not much you can do to fight against it. While people say things happen for a reason, people resent not knowing what that reason is. Life is not about getting things back to the way they were, but to evolve from hardships and achieve a better life. The issues that come to your present state means you are ready for a better one. Like a cat that moves on from one life to the next, regard your struggles as a chance for a new beginning.

"Exercises are like prose, whereas yoga is the poetry of movements. Once you understand the grammar of yoga; you can write your poetry of movements."

Amit Ray

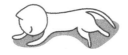

Practicing yoga should be routine, but the poses you perform should not. As a novice, it is mandatory to seek guidance from instructors on how to practice yoga, just as how kittens learn from their mothers how to hunt and pounce. Once you master a set of skills and understand how your body moves and strengthens, you can express yourself through your own movements. Yoga will become your body's language.

"Mountain pose teaches us, literally, how to stand on our own two feet, teaching us to root ourselves into the earth. Our bodies become a connection between heaven and earth."

Carol Krucoff

When you stand, understand your importance. Let the scattered thoughts in your head slip away from you as you face the world and acknowledge your presence in the world. You are strong. You are calm. You are here and you are living. Approach the world like a lion and roar!

"Yoga is the perfect opportunity to be curious about who you are."

Jason Crandell

Life is confusing. You may not know which career path you want to take, what you're looking for in a partner, whether you're ready for a family beyond your kitty or need more adventure. Yoga allows you to take time to sit down with yourself and get answers from deep within you. Meditate on what you want, breathe in desire and breathe out anxieties. Discover yourself.

"For me, yoga is not just a workout—it's about working on yourself."

Mary Glover

Whether you find a "spiritual journey" unnecessary or cheesy, when you practice yoga, you are doing more than balancing on one leg and stretching your muscles. You are taking an active part in bringing peace and quiet into your day to clear your mind. That in itself will calm your mind every day, and you will come to discover who you really are.

"Between stimulus and response, there is a space. In that space is our power to choose our response. In our response lies our growth and our freedom."

Viktor E. Frankl

There will be opportunities reaching out to you and how you choose to respond to them will speak to who you are. Are you a curious kitten or a scaredy cat? There can be growth in accepting a new passage, but there can also be freedom from rejecting the wrong pathway. In the space between opportunity and decision, take advantage of self-reflection and gain power in your choice.

"Yoga is a balancing factor, a substratum across all of your life, so you do not get shifted in one direction or another. It gives you freshness, gives you light, recharges your batteries. You become a stable person. You realize what balance is, what sukha is, what contentment is, what joy is."

Birjoo Mehta

Yoga as a practiced routine should be regarded as the anchoring point of clarity for yourself. It is time that you meditate to step back from your issues and resolve them. It is an exercise to sustain health, to realize your body is greater than you ever imagined. It is a time to face yourself, to realize your mind is stronger than its demons. It is a time to be alive!

"Yoga is not about touching your toes, it is what you learn on the way down."

Jigar Gor

People become preoccupied with achieving perfection rather than acknowledging the lessons they learn along the way. For every mistake you make, you gain more wisdom, like an alley cat veteran who knows how to work the town. Who you are when you have to face obstacles is a greater life lesson than when you accomplish them. Take your self-discovery slowly. Do not be so quick to rush this journey.

"Yoga is possible for anybody who really wants it. Yoga is universal. But don't approach yoga with a business mind looking for worldly gain."

Sri Krishna Pattabhi Jois

When you bring yoga into your life, remind yourself that the gain should be entirely personal. You should not be doing yoga to look good in front of others, to show off skill in flexibility in front of your cat, or to preach cliché wisdom to friends. Practice yoga with the sole purpose of bettering yourself, both physically and mentally. You are your only concern. But okay, maybe you can show off in front of your cat.

"Corpse Pose sounds like no big deal, right? Then what's so difficult about this spiritualized snooze? Forget about getting your feet behind your head. Just try lying still for ten minutes. With nothing left to do, you're finally forced to come face to face with yourself."

Edward Vilga

The true test of the spirit is to not take advantage of falling asleep on yourself to avoid confronting your deepest thoughts, both literally and figuratively. This is a moment to lie still on the earth and face your fears, be they rejection or failure or death. Are you satisfied with your life and how things are? Wake yourself up from passive living and revive your passion. Become alive again.

"While doing yoga we are more ourselves, and more than ourselves."

Valerie Jeremijenko

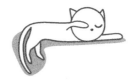

"Be at least as interested in what goes on inside you as what happens outside. If you get the inside right, the outside will fall into place."

Eckhart Tolle

Become less preoccupied with what life brings you and negative influences from forces you cannot control. Focus your observations to what improvements you are making in your own flexibility and strength, whether it is from your muscles becoming more limber or your brain finding more answers to deal with stress. Fine-tune yourself. Every day the cat stretches its limbs and its mind to keep itself in shape.

"Your task is not to seek for love, but merely to seek and find all the barriers within yourself that you have built against it."

Helen Schucman

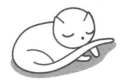

To accept love into your heart is to realize where your insecurities lie. Happiness is not something that comes with ease, but with the motivation to overcome your demons. When you pinpoint what you consider negative in yourself, you can begin the process of healing and understanding that you are a beautiful, complex person, worthy of loving yourself and others.

"Don't ask yourself what the world needs; ask yourself what makes you come alive. And then go and do that. Because what the world needs is people who have come alive."

Howard Thurman

Those who have happiness spread happiness. Do not put such pressuring weight on your shoulders to solve the world's problems. What makes you happy? What do you call a beautiful day, one to share with others? What invokes love in your heart to spread around? Ask yourself what makes you smile. It could be as simple as hearing your kitty friend purr you to sleep.

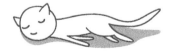

God
&
Spirituality

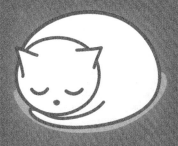

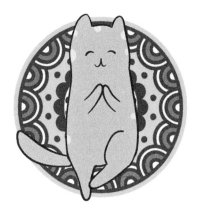

Tree Pose

Stand up straight. Lay your left foot on your right thigh. Be careful not to lose your balance. Clasp your hands together in Namaste at chest level, as if to begin prayer. Hold. Switch legs after a few breaths. Try not to stumble.

"I am standing on my own altar; the poses are my prayers."

B.K.S. Iyengar

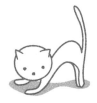

Begin your routine by understanding that your body is using yoga as a form of expression, as a means of communicating its needs and desires as it reaches out for a challenge each day. You're not a lazy cat; you're a person ready to evolve. As you stand on your yoga mat, stretch up to the skies and speak!

"You are an aperture through which the universe is looking at and exploring itself."

Alan Wilson Watts

Your greatness is to be discovered. Allow yourself to be a channel for energy to flow through you and inspire change within yourself. Just as how you welcome your kitty friend to caress you with warmth, welcome the universe into your heart. Let yourself be seen and loved and you will shine even brighter.

"The aspirant would do well to avoid those 'spiritual teachers' who delight in pointing out the evils of the world. These are immature egos attempting to discard their own negativities by projecting them onto others. The true yogi is one who is like a lion with himself, always striving to eradicate that which shadows his inner light, and like a lamb with others, always striving to see their inner light, no matter how dense may be the clouds that hide it. He is the king of the jungle of his world. He hides from no one and seeks escape from nothing."

Prem Prakash

After dark, all cats are leopards. Even if you understand that there is evil in the world, do not let the unknown intimidate you. Sometimes troubles are smaller than they seem and sometimes warnings from others are their own projected fears. Stand brave against the world by having confidence in yourself. You are strong and capable of anything. Do not let the shadows fool you.

"What we're trying to do in yoga is to create a union, and so to deepen a yoga pose is to actually increase the union of the pose, not necessarily put your leg around your head."

Rodney Yee

Flexibility is an ideal you should want to achieve, yes, but it shouldn't be your only goal. Getting to know your body and how it moves or where it shivers is the step to reuniting yourself with your temple. Observe the unique traits of your skin and your muscles. See where you are strong and which parts of you remain fertile and soft. Revel in your own wonder.

"If I'm losing balance in a pose, I stretch higher and God reaches down to steady me. It works every time, and not just in yoga."

Terri Guillemets

There is no shame in reaching out to a higher being to give you a sense of protection. As a spiritual journey, yoga allows you to find guidance from heaven when you don't feel balanced in your position. Do not panic and fall to the ground. Reach out. Someone will help you.

"Crying is one of the highest devotional songs. One who knows crying, knows spiritual practice. If you can cry with a pure heart, nothing else compares to such a prayer. Crying includes all the principles of Yoga."

Kripalvanandji

No one is suggesting you wail like a street cat at midnight, but understand that crying can be a cathartic coping mechanism. Never be ashamed of having an emotional reaction to the outside world. Look at crying as a cleansing of the spirit, ridding the negative energy from you as you cry for your soul to be restored. Crying doesn't solve anything, but it does release you from tension.

"What yoga philosophy and all the great Buddhist teachings tells us is that solidity is a creation of the ordinary mind and that there never was anything permanent to begin with that we could hold on to. Life would be much easier and substantially less painful if we lived with the knowledge of impermanence as the only constant."

Donna Farhi

Rid yourself of any attachment you have with possessions. Things that hold true meaning have no tangible surface to grab onto, like love and happiness. Pick up your cat and marvel at its beautiful existence and bask in the affection you have for it. Live knowing good comes from within you, not an object in your hand.

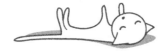

"The harmonizing of opposing forces is a key aspect of yoga — hot energy is united with cool energy, strong with soft, and masculine with feminine."

Tara Fraser

Take in the ferocity of a tiger with the grace of an alley cat and you'll find yourself harmonizing masculinity and femininity within yourself. Yoga demands a sense of balance between your flexibility and your strength, which you will learn to control and challenge as a united force.

"When you live your life with an appreciation of coincidences and their meanings, you connect with the underlying field of infinite possibilities."

Deepak Chopra

Things happen for a reason, but there an infinite amount of them to choose from. When you start to appreciate the small happenstances of life and put an optimistic outlook on them, you can open yourself to living carefree, like a cat who remembers it has nine lives. The chance of something great happening is always likely if you open yourself to a wonderful day each day.

"If you want to find God, hang out in the space between your thoughts."

Alan Cohen

There are answers inside you, real deep, past all the anxieties and lurking in the silence between your thoughts. Breathe. Tune in to yourself and listen to your conscious speak. God can be the whisper in your mind or the purr rumbling from your heart to enjoy the moment. Yoga is the anchor to your thoughts, reminding you to stop and observe the world around you. You might just see something enlightening.

"Inhale, and God approaches you. Hold the inhalation, and God remains with you. Exhale, and you approach God. Hold the exhalation, and surrender to God."

Tirumalai Krishnamacharya

For every breath you breathe, you are going through a spiritual connection. Let it be a constant reminder of your precious life: take in the world with each inhale and devote your life to everything around you with each exhale. When you lie with your kitty, appreciate the breaths you share. This is your union with universal life.

"What each of us believes in is up to us, but life is impossible without believing in something."

Kentetsu Takamori

When you bring yoga into your life, people will want to force their spirituality onto you, but you define your own spirituality, whether it lies in a higher power or solely in yourself. Enwrap yourself in the world around you, be it nature or the love within your community. Find something to believe in. When you practice yoga, you are searching for union not only in yourself, but with the universe as well. And if all else fails, find solace in your cat!

"Yoga is not a religion. It is a science, science of well-being, science of youthfulness, science of integrating body, mind and soul."

Amit Ray

While there is nothing wrong with finding a sense of spirituality in practicing yoga, yoga is also a personal journey, one that shows your playfulness and your contentment, like a kitten stretching before its morning play. Consider the focus of your concern to be yourself as you discover what you want out of life. Do you want to reinvent yourself or do you just want some peace as you cuddle with your kitty?

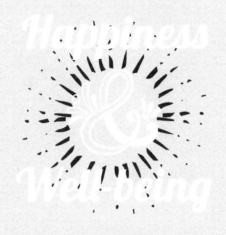

Happiness & Well-being

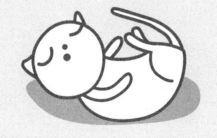

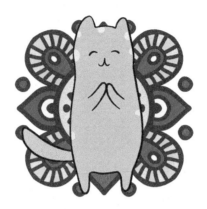

Mountain Pose

Stand up straight with your legs together or at an even stance. Straighten your shoulders and on an inhale, raise your arms straight above your head. Extend your backbone and entire body up, stretch as far as you can. Make sure your arms are straight and parallel with each other. Reach and hold, without lifting your heels off the ground.

"That's exactly how it is in yoga. The places where you have the most resistance are actually the places that are going to be the areas of the greatest liberation."

Rodney Yee

Don't be a scaredy cat about your challenges! You will be faced with resistance and you will be tempted to build a brick wall of insecurities before your goal, but you have to believe in yourself. Yoga is about molding you into the image you want to display. Don't give up when you are so close to reaching your goals. Liberate yourself and go for it!

"When you listen to yourself, everything comes naturally. It comes from inside, like a kind of will to do something. Try to be sensitive. That is yoga."

Petri Räisänen

As you fine-tune your skills in meditation, you will learn to listen to yourself and discover where your true nature lies. Just as how you pay close attention to hear your kitty purr, pay attention to what makes you truly content. Be sensitive to your honest wishes. Let yoga give you the opportunity to see yourself and be happy with who you are.

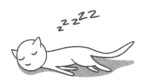

"I think the time is right for yoga. We really are living in a very complex time — a time of great turmoil and change. Yoga is a good antidote to all that. It is almost like music in a way; there's no end to it."

Sting

These days, it might seem like the world is in constant peril, whether it's the constant reel of tragedies on your newsfeed or overwhelming personal matters. You may want to hide away with your cat and never step outside again, but instead take this opportunity to let yoga make you strong. Bring control back into your life by disciplining your mind and body every day. Shut out complexities from your spirit.

"Yoga is the fountain of youth. You're only as young as your spine is flexible."

Bob Harper

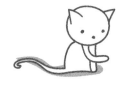

It seems like cats never age, do they? Take a lesson from your feline companion and regard flexibility as key to your nature. Stretch your body each morning to brace the day. Curl your limbs to find comfort in the most unlikely positions. Let your body adapt to the world around you. Even as a cat falls, it twists itself to land on its feet. Your youth lies in your flexibility.

"Yoga is invigoration in relaxation. Freedom in routine. Confidence through self-control. Energy within and energy without."

Ymber Delecto

It might be a difficult journey, but when you climb over the hill of dreading your yoga routine (because it will happen), there will be a euphoric sensation every time you finish your poses. The normalcy will bring you comfort, the steady progress will show, and your energy will become infinite. Like a cat ready to play, you'll leap over any feat to purrfect harmony.

"Better indeed is knowledge than mechanical practice. Better than knowledge is meditation. But better still is surrender of attachment to results, because there follows immediate peace."

Bhagavad Gita

"It is my conviction that there is no way to peace—peace is the way."

Thich Nhat Hanh

To achieve peace, you must embody it. Change comes from within. Before you can change the world, you need to sit with yourself and find peace for you. Be selfishly persistent in finding your own happiness, so that you can go to others, glowing with confidence. Find peace within yourself and you will only breed peace in relationships with others.

"If we learn to open our hearts, anyone, including the people who drive us crazy, can be our teacher."

Pema Chödrön

There are lessons to be learned from everyone. When getting to know your cat, you had to go through trials and tribulations to understand their character, so that you both could live in harmony. Well, the same goes for people who bring you conflict. Open yourself to compromise. Meditate on what you can improve that can bring the best out of the both of you.

To achieve peace requires hard work. It takes dedication to restore relationships and to develop good self-esteem, but this work will be fruitful. The routine of taking care of others to receive kindness will become natural. Just as how taking care of your cat is second-nature to you, with its snuggles being a much-appreciated reward, work for peace and you'll rarely have to deal with war.

Waiting for the world to fix itself will leave you dead. You are your own change. Make the differences you want and abide to your principles. Your happiness relies on you and should never be dependent on others. Allow the universe to be kind to you, but never expect it. What you give controls what you take.

"Through the practices of yoga, we discover that concern for the happiness and well-being of others, including animals, must be an essential part of our own quest for happiness and well-being. The fork can be a powerful weapon of mass destruction or a tool to create peace on Earth."

Sharon Gannon

No one needs to tell you that you can find happiness in the well-being of your cat(s), but the same goes for people. The principle of finding joy in the happiness of others is sometimes difficult to practice with petty demons such as envy and resentment, but when you open your heart to live through the success of others, you will find peace in seeing someone else's smile.

"Undisturbed calmness of mind is attained by cultivating friendliness toward the happy, compassion for the unhappy, delight in the virtuous, and indifference toward the wicked."

Patanjali

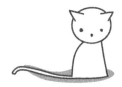

There is a purity in a kitten's affection that you should display to all your neighbors, and for your enemies, reject them with the cool indifference of a mature feline. Spread joy and you will receive it tenfold. Reject negativity from your life and you will cleanse your pathway to happiness. Mark standards for yourself that fulfill you. Settle for nothing less.

"I've learned that people will forget what you said, people will forget what you did, but people will never forget how you made them feel."

Maya Angelou

Humble your ego by reminding yourself that your importance lies in how you treat others, not in how they remember you. Yoga keeps your ego in check as you center yourself to meditate on yourself, but express positivity to others. What makes you love? You love your cat not because of what it does but because of how it makes you feel. Spread this love. Make the world feel warmth from your heart.

"The things that matter most in our lives are not fantastic or grand. They are the moments when we touch one another."

Jack Kornfield

Why do you love your cat? Because it can perform miracles and give you everything you ever wanted? No. Because your cat comforts you, reminds you that the world isn't always bad. The same peace you get cuddling with your fluffy loved one should be the same peace you get through yoga—the reminder that the relationships we form with the world are what bring light in our life.

"Live with intention. Walk to the edge. Listen hard. Practice wellness. Play with abandon. Laugh. Choose with no regret. Appreciate your friends. Continue to learn. Do what you love. Live as if this is all there is."

Mary Radmacher

Enjoy life! Yoga is about connecting with the world by embracing your own spirit! Play with your kitty; stretch with your best friend and relax in the bed comforters afterwards. Remind yourself that you love and live for those reasons. Life is all around you for you to enjoy, so get up and smile!

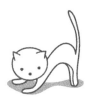

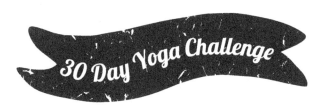

30 Day Yoga Challenge

By Paige Hodges

In this book you have been introduced to several beneficial yoga poses and inspired by the words of yogi masters. We've learned that cats make excellent yoga teachers and they have much to teach us. Now it's time to challenge ourselves. Let's take what we have learned and put it into action.

My feline companion Pippy and I invite you to a 30 Day Yoga Challenge. Pippy is a master feline yogini and I have studied under her tutelage since she was a kitten. She has taught me much and continues to do so. Our yoga challenge is meant to be fun and there are no steadfast rules, only guidelines. No matter what your fitness level, our challenge will meet you where you're at in your yoga journey.

If you've never done yoga, great! You are in for a treat and we are so excited for you. If you already have a practice, then this challenge will help you amp up your practice another notch. You already know that a yoga practice is well worth your time and this challenge will give you the opportunity to explore the next level. Please note that the instructions and advice presented are in no way intended as a substitute for medical counseling. As with any physical program, consult your medical professional of choice if you have any concerns. Remember, it's up to you to take responsibility for your body and well being and you know best what you need.

This challenge is not a one size fits all. We won't tell you exactly what to do but we will guide you. Part of the challenge is discovering what is appropriate for your body right now. Although we will all work differently, we will all reap healthy benefits for our mind, body, and soul.

One of the aims of this challenge is to form a yoga habit. Practicing yoga every day for 30 days will help us to do so. There are different schools of thought about how long it takes to form a habit, but 30 days is definitely in the ball park. The key is commitment, setting an intention, and following through. The Yoga Sutras of Patanjali tell us in verse 1:14: "This practice becomes firmly rooted when it is cultivated skillfully and continuously for a long time."

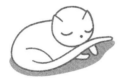

Here are the guidelines:

Set your intention to practice yoga every day.

Aim for at least 30 minutes a day and if you want to practice longer, all the better. If you are new to yoga and 10-15 minutes is all you can complete, that's ok, but aim to work up to 30 minutes by the end of the challenge.

3

You can practice in your home or in a yoga class. You may even prefer a little of both. If you practice at home, designate a special place that you can call your own that is free of distraction. Preferably make it a space that is spacious and soothing to your eyes.

4

Decide which yoga poses you will practice each day and make a list of some new or challenging poses you would like to work on. This may take some research. If you are new to yoga and don't have any idea which poses to practice, consider taking a beginner yoga class or checking out an online yoga class or yoga DVD. Several poses have also been mentioned in this book, so choose one or two that are appropriate for your fitness level.

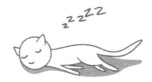

Whether you are new to yoga or a long time practitioner, remember that some days it may be enough to just lie on your back with your feet up against the wall and breathe deeply. We don't always have to practice strenuous poses. Remember to listen to your body.

Make it fun. Reward yourself each day you practice. Get a special calendar and document each day with a colorful sticker or star when you have finished your practice. Another idea is to reward yourself at the end of each week with a little luxury of your choice.

Take care of your body. Remember to breathe and eat nourishing foods.

And most importantly, observe the cats in your life. They are our best teachers!

Pippy, The Feline Yogini, loves being of service to humans and helping them improve their yoga practices. She is very intuitive and her wish is that her purr-ful insights will inspire you to succeed. I now leave you with a special message from Pippy:

Greetings Humans!

Are you excited? Are you ready to get started on The 30 Day Yoga Challenge? I love the opportunity to work with humans because it has taught me patience and acceptance. No wonder we felines are such great yogis. We are constantly given the opportunity to cultivate equanimity. And we do it well, don't we?

First of all let's talk cats! Keep in mind that you will get so much more out of the yoga challenge if you seriously study us cats. Don't just stare at us admiringly but really study us. If you don't have a cat companion, observe your friend's cat or go visit a shelter or rescue group. The cats there will love the company and you may find yourself adding a new member to your family.

You may be wondering, "What must I look for when I observe your superior species, Pippy?" So glad you asked and I'm happy to enlighten you. Spend at least a good ten minutes simply watching us. Notice our deep breathing and how we make the most out of each stretch we take. Also notice how we are perfectly content to just sit and be. I would give you more things to look out for but it will behoove you to figure it out on your own as that is part of your yoga practice journey.

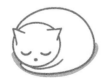

Speaking of journeys, this challenge is all about the journey dear humans. You humans are always rushing around frantically trying to get somewhere. There is nowhere to go! That's the secret! Because when you get there, you will want to go somewhere else! Right? Enjoy where your yoga practice is right now. This does not mean that you will not strive for more but that you are grateful for where you are at the present time.

Be aware of excuses. You humans love excuses. "My Netflix queue is full and I must catch up; I am too tired!; I can't find my yoga pants! blah blah blah" The list goes on and on. You are responsible for setting your priorities. That may mean watching less TV or prying yourself away from Facebook, but it's up to you and you only to make sure to find the time.

Don't underestimate the value of sleep. Too many of you humans are sleep deprived and wake up numerous times during the night. Some of you wake up in the middle of your slumber to check your smart phones! Yoga will help you sleep better and maybe you will eventually sleep as well as us cats. I personally like to get a good night's sleep so I can rise and shine extra early and start the day with a hearty meal about an hour before the sun comes up. A regular yoga practice will help you sleep well too so you are ready to jump out of bed and into the kitchen at the earliest hour possible. After feeding us kitties, you might find the wee hours of the morning are a great time to engage in your yoga practice.

When practicing a yoga asana (asana is the Sanskrit word for pose) don't make such a big deal about what you look like in the asana. Just because the lithe young kitten down the street looks a certain way while doing a pose doesn't mean that every cat has to try to emulate her. The same thing applies to you humans. Show confidence while doing the poses and compete with only yourself.

Does your cat like to practice with you? Does she take a place on your yoga mat as soon as you roll it out? Does she supervise you while you try to master a particularly challenging pose? Good! She's trying to help you. Let her!

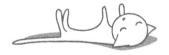

As you move along in your yoga practice, many things will happen. I'm excited to tell you about them and how your life and your cat's lives will improve. You will develop strength. Strength comes in handy when you have to move the couch to fetch a lost cat toy, transport kitties to the vet in a carrier, or lift large boxes of cat litter down from store shelves. You will become more flexible. Scooping litter boxes requires a lot of squatting and bending. Having a human who can keep up with this task is very important. You may also be required to contort your body in several different types of positions while sleeping each night in order to accommodate where we kitties like to rest our heads.

Yoga helps you develop patience. For example in our household, some days I like to get on the kitchen cabinets even though I know they are a "no no" place. But I can't help it as they are so temping and the view is so magnificent. I do not need to be spoken to in a loud obnoxious voice or be threatened with a water bottle. No, I need a human with patience to wait until I'm good and ready to get down. My humans have not quite mastered this but I trust they will get there. Yoga also helps you be more intuitive so you can anticipate your kitty's needs.

Why should any feline have to beg for a snack or anything else for that matter? The more intuitive a human is, the better they can serve the felines in their life.

Last but not least, I will address a question that humans often ask me. Why is downward-facing dog pose not called downward-facing cat pose and how do you feel about that? Downward-facing dog was originally meant to be called downward-facing cat until the dog lobby invested millions in making the name change. (This was news to me but my conspiracy-loving cat companions swear it's true!) At any rate, it doesn't really matter to us cats. We know that no species can "downward cat" quite like us.

Best of luck with the 30 Day Yoga Challenge! Remember: Pippy here supports you 110% and so do the feline yogis in your life.

Meow and Namaste, dear humans!

The great feline spirit in me salutes the beautiful human spirit in you!

Love,
Pippy, The Feline Yogini

Closing

By Paige Hodges

Cats make yoga look easy, don't they? They come out of the womb enlightened while we humans just stagger along pitifully trying to figure it out all out. But fear not, there's still hope for our species. We can master yoga too and our feline companions can help show us the way.

Why do we find cats so enchanting? Cats have a complicated yet fascinating history in regards to their relationship with us. The ancient Egyptians worshipped them as gods and it's often joked that cats have never forgotten this. Whether cats find this funny or true, well, we'd have to ask them. The medieval church saw them as a symbol of witchcraft and persecuted them as agents of the devil. However, cats made a comeback in the Age of Enlightenment and were welcomed into the homes of royalty and the upper classes. Most recently we have seen a resurgence in the cat's popularity. A whole segment of our society just can't get enough of cats.

Perhaps the period we live in will go down in history as not only a time when cats were passionately loved and admired, but an era when we finally started taking advantage of what we could learn about the art of yoga from them. Whether you are about to embark on a yoga practice for the first time or you've been practicing for years, observe and study how your kitty approaches the practice. Be open to something new and let your feline guide you. You won't be disappointed.

Cats are natural yogis for more reasons than their superb flexibility. Yes those flexible spines they possess are enviable, but that's just part of what they have to offer. Most importantly, cats know how to live in the moment. They don't worry about the past or the future because they always focus on the here and now. Felines take it one day at a time and trust that their needs will be met. Granted, we humans meet most of their needs, but the point is they trust that we will!

Cats don't compare themselves to other cats and certainly not to humans. Each feline knows they are perfect exactly the way they were created. They know that beauty comes in all different forms and we each have something unique to offer the world. They don't covet another cat's catnip stash or kitty condo. "Keeping up with the Joneses" is not on their radar because the Joneses are status quo and a cat would never succumb to coveting anything that didn't celebrate their individuality.

Cats are fearless. They have no qualms about trying out a new pose and will contort themselves in any direction if it's fun and feels good. How they look in a particular pose is of no interest to them, but how it makes them feel is! They don't hesitate to crawl into small spaces like underneath the sofa or a house guest's lap. They are not shy when it comes to finding out what's it's like to hang from the living room drapes. They think nothing of exploring the tops of kitchen cabinets, computer

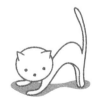

keyboards while in use, or any type of box or sink. While these antics may not be practical (or even achievable) for us humans, it's still a great reminder to have fun and bring a sense of playfulness to our yoga practice. Cats are adventurous and love taking risks, characteristics that are essential to all yogis.

Cats can sit and meditate for hours without moving. Even though kitties may look still and content, they are always aware of their surroundings. If you doubt this, bring out the can opener or open a cupboard where there may be some food and a cat will come running. Meditation is not sleep, it is a practice of concentrated attention to aid in spiritual growth. Cats definitely have this down!

Cats don't make excuses. They find time to practice yoga and spend quality time with themselves. Some might argue that cats are selfish, but are they really? Is it selfish to take care of our well being and health? They know that if they don't nurture their spirit, they will have nothing to give back to the human companions in their lives.

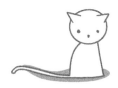

Cats know the importance of deep breathing. Humans pay lip service to the concept, but how many of us really relish in the healing power of our own breath? Too often we take mostly small breaths resulting in shallow breathing. This type of breathing adds more stress to our already chaotic lives. Cats on the other hand take long deep breaths. How often do you see a stressed out cat? Even when a kitty is stalking her prey, whether it be real or imaginary, her breath is deep, full, and focused.

A cat's movements are always brilliantly choreographed, whether they are pouncing, strutting, or at play chasing their tail. Their flexible spines allow enlightening energy to move through them quite effortlessly. Each graceful movement has intention, purpose, and commitment. The feline's elegant movements are in tune with the music of life. It's as if they dance to a tune that we humans are not privy to or maybe we could be if only we stilled ourselves long enough to listen.

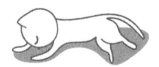

Cats are aware that life is constantly changing and they go with the flow like brilliant improvisational artists. Cats are little Zen masters with a powerful presence. Cats don't just exist. They have mastered the art of living and are connoisseurs of strength and balance. They naturally create balance in their lives and don't have to think about it, as it is second nature to them. Cats are tantamount to observing a brilliant work of art. You constantly see something different and the learning never stops.

Living with cats is a privilege and lucky us who have the honor of doing so! Let's take advantage of our good fortune and roll out those yoga mats. It's time to start practicing some serious downward-facing cat poses! Are you up to it? Your cat certainly is and you wouldn't want to squander an opportunity to study with a yoga master, would you? May the blessings of yoga touch both you and your cat.

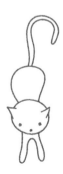

CPSIA information can be obtained at www.ICGtesting.com
Printed in the USA
BVOW11s1933060116

431948BV00005B/5/P